Plant-Based Diets:

Embracing the Power of Plants for a Healthy Life

By

LENA R JOHNSON

COPYRIGHT

All rights reserved. No part of this publication may be reproduced, distributed, or transmitted in any form or by any means, including photocopying, recording, or other electronic or mechanical methods, without the prior written permission of the publisher, except in the case of brief quotations embodied in critical reviews and certain other noncommercial uses permitted by copyright law.

This publication is protected by copyright law and international treaties. Unauthorized reproduction or distribution of this publication, or any portion of it, may result in severe civil and criminal penalties and will be prosecuted to the maximum extent possible under the law.

For permissions requests, please contact:

Email: Johnsonlenar11@gmail.com

TABLE OF CONTENT

INTRODUCTION

Greetings from the fascinating and revolutionary realm of plant-based diets! We cordially urge you to go on a transformative journey with this all-inclusive guide, "Plant-Based Diets: Embracing the Power of Plants for a Healthy Life," which will not only fuel not just your body but also the earth and your soul. Making the switch to a plant-based diet is an influential decision motivated by an aim for improved well-being, a sustainable future, and a kind relationship with all living things.

'The Revolution Based on Plants'

Plant-based diets have gained popularity recently as a global phenomenon that draws visitors from all backgrounds. It's a wave of change, a philosophy, and a way of life rather than merely a diet. It's about selecting foods that satisfy our cravings while also being in line with our morals and the demands of the environment.

'Your Well-being, Your Money' You are investing in your health and well-being when you decide to learn more about plant-based nutrition. Learn how your food can be your most powerful medicine on this trip. There are several well-established advantages to a plant-based diet, ranging from lowering the risk of chronic diseases to reaching and maintaining a healthy weight.

A plant-based diet consists primarily or exclusively of meals derived from plants. Diverse interpretations and applications exist for the term "plant-based diet" It is sometimes misunderstood as a vegan diet, which excludes all animal products. For others, a plant-based diet consists primarily of plant foods such as fruits, vegetables, whole grains, nuts, and legumes; nevertheless, they may occasionally eat dairy, fish, or meat. Healthy whole foods are the main emphasis of a plant-based diet as opposed to processed meals. Raw vegan meals have become a popular and health-conscious alternative in a world where nutritional choices are as varied as the people who make them.

PLANT-BASED DIETS

Raw vegan meals, which embrace the unadulterated nature of uncooked plant-based foods, provide a delicious approach to fueling the body with nutrient-dense goodness. This piece delves into the appealing realm of raw vegan cuisine, emphasizing its health advantages, adaptability in the kitchen, and the delight of indulging in raw, plant-based dishes.

PART 1

Chapter 1

A Personal Journey Towards A Plant-Based, Whole-Foods Diet

Upon joining Kaiser Permanente (KP) in 2003, two of my very first patients were Robert and Rose Anne Park. They got married and lived in several US locations before settling in Bakersfield, California, to raise their family. They had first met at a United Service Organization (USO) dance in Ocean side, California. Mr. Park, who was involved in the church, was appointed Pastor Robert. He frequently served as a volunteer Sunday school teacher and

held courses for recently married couples. Mr. Park did not prioritize his health; like many others whose life's mission is to help others. He battled to control his weight and was prescribed several medications, including insulin, for diabetes and high blood pressure.

Mr. Park emailed me in the spring of 2012 to report that he had seen blood in his urine and to inquire as to whether this was cause for alarm.

I told him we would diagnose the issue and ordered a computed tomography scan of his kidneys.

His kidneys did not exhibit any concerning results from the scan. It did, however, reveal many tumors in his pancreatic and liver. Following additional examinations and biopsies, Mr. Park was diagnosed with metastatic pancreatic cancer. He saw an oncologist, who informed him of his dismal prognosis, and he decided to stop receiving any therapy. Thanks to his trust in Jesus Christ, he was able to live out his final days fearlessly after enrolling in hospice care. A few weeks later, he passed away at home in the company of his cherished family.

His wife visited me a few weeks following his passing. My initial observation was that Mrs. Park had shed a significant amount of weight. I surmised that it was due to the strain of her husband's illness and the sorrow of his passing. When our meeting came to a close, she asked if I would commit to doing something for her. Specifically, she requested me to read Joel Fuhrman, MD's book Eat to Live.

She added that following her husband's diagnosis, their son started looking for information on how to lower his own risk as well as the reasons behind the development of his father's pancreatic cancer. His studies led their family to adopt a plant-based diet, which improved their general health and helped them lose weight. "I know it's too late for

Robert, but maybe this information can help someone else," she said to me before we left the visit. I had to tell myself that, despite my skepticism about the possibility that diet could influence cancer risk, I had learned very little about nutrition during my residency and medical school. I struggled with my weight over the first few years after joining KP, having gained about 6.75 kg (15 lb) and experiencing sporadic gout attacks. I had to make a big choice after reading Eat to Live, The China Study, and other books detailing the science behind a whole-foods-based, plant-based diet's health advantages. Do I disregard all the study and scientific data I now have about the advantages of a plant-based diet for health? Or was I prepared to confront my ego and my present perspective on nutrition and health? To address that, I reluctantly decided to give a plant-based diet a try.

I started out removing everything dairy and animal goods save eggs and fish because I was unwilling to commit completely overnight. After a month, I felt healthier, slept better, had more energy, and had lost 4.5 kg (10 lb).

After seeing the results, I set a goal for myself to go a month without eating any animal products and only eat plant-based foods. I was down from my high school weight by the end of the month, and I had stopped having gout attacks. I adopted this idea into my medical practice and urged my patients to attempt a whole-food, plant-based diet because I had personally experienced its advantages. The goal of a whole-food, plant-based diet is to consume as many nutrient-dense plant foods as possible while limiting processed foods, fats, and animal products (such as dairy and eggs). It is often low in fat and promotes a diet high in fruits, vegetables (cooked or raw), beans, peas, lentils, soybeans, seeds, and nuts (in smaller amounts). While many proponents of whole foods, plant-based diets are vegan and abstain from all animal products, another popular approach is to be "flexitarian," meaning that you occasionally eat modest amounts of dairy and animal protein.

When I told my patients about my own experience and that I would be closely monitoring them, many of them were open to trying a diet that was primarily plant-based.

The outcomes shocked me. Many patients were able to cut back or stop taking the years-long prescriptions for diabetes and hypertension in a matter of weeks. They informed me they would have stopped taking their meds long ago if they had known that all it took was a simple change in diet. Many, however, had never been informed that this was an option and hence thought that medication was the only way to manage these diseases. I found that "prescribing" drugs was a more fulfilling professional experience than writing prescriptions for several different medications for my chronic disease patients.

Chapter 2

Health Advantages of Plant-Based Diet

A plant-based diet has numerous potential health advantages, such as more effective weight control

According to research, people who eat mostly plant-based diets typically have lower incidences of obesity, diabetes, and heart disease, as well as a lower body mass index (BMI) than people who eat meat. Diets based mostly on plants are high in water content from fruits and vegetables, fiber, and complex carbs. People may feel fuller for longer and consume more energy while they are sleeping as a result of this. According to a 2018 study, treating obesity with a plant-based diet proved successful.

75 obese or overweight participants in the study were divided into two groups: those who continued eating meat

in their regular diet or those who adopted a vegan diet. Only the vegan group demonstrated a noteworthy 14.33-pound (6.5-kilogram) weight loss after 4 months.

In contrast to the group that ate a typical diet with meat, the plant-based vegan group experienced improvements in insulin sensitivity and reduced fat mass. Vegans had the lowest average body mass index(BMI), followed by lacto-ovo vegetarians (those who eat dairy and eggs) and pescatarians (those who eat fish but no other meat), according to a 2009 survey of over 60,000 people. Nonvegetarians were the group with the higher average BMI.

Difficulties In Changing Medicine Culture

When I share my newfound perspective with my colleagues, I usually get the following responses, even though many of my patients have been open to my advice regarding nutrition: "I don't have the time to talk to patients about nutrition," "I don't feel I know counsel patients on lifestyle," "Nutrition has little to no impact on health and chronic disease," or just "I could never give up eating meat." Their answers demonstrate the enormous obstacles that lie ahead in transforming the medical establishment to prioritize lifestyle medicine and a "nutrition first" strategy for illness prevention and treatment.

Physicians may now access an increasing amount of resources to educate them about the role diet plays in both the prevention and treatment of disease. You may go to a conference on nutrition, finish an online course like the Cornell credential in Plant-Based Nutrition, get board-certified by the American College of Lifestyle Medicine, or browse online materials like Michael Greger, MD's website. Regardless of the tools employed, all medical professionals should aim to become knowledgeable about nutrition science and research to enable their patients to take the required actions to take charge of and improve their health.

For my medical colleagues who claim, "I could never give up meat," I think it is our duty as doctors to advise patients on the foods that will best support their overall health and well-being, even if we don't always heed our counsel. This would be comparable to doctors who smoke but advise and support their patients to give up smoking. Our healthcare issue may be solved if disease prevention and treatment use a nutrition-first approach.

It is concerning because, over the past ten years, US healthcare prices have increased faster than inflation, housing and food expenditures, and other costs. More than any other nation, we spend more than $3 trillion annually on health care, but our life expectancy and clinical results are not among the finest in the world. Over 70% of Americans are overweight or obese, according to the CDC. There is a direct correlation between the rising incidence of diabetes, heart disease, and cancer and the rising rates of obesity. There is no way to continue this way, and no practical measures have been taken to stop the cost of living increases. While technological, medical, and personalized treatment advancements are encouraging, I think they will likely drive up rather than lower the overall cost of healthcare. Many individuals will still struggle in the meanwhile under our present healthcare delivery system, particularly those with limited access to healthcare and financial means.

Furthermore, there is little to no financial incentive to alter the present diagnose-and-treat strategy under the conventional fee-for-service reimbursement model in the healthcare industry.

In fee-for-service practice, doctors frequently complain that they "eat what you kill" in the medical field because their compensation is based solely on productivity and only covers in-person patient care, interventions, and treatments. Sandeep Jauhar, MD, a cardiologist and New York Times columnist describes firsthand the financial hardships and frequently mismatched financial incentives that physicians face in fee-for-service medicine in his book Doctored: The Disillusionment of an American Physician.

Healthy individuals usually don't need much medical attention. Therefore, when healthy patients choose not to seek care, physicians are not compensated under a fee-for-service approach. Pay is no longer correlated with production in a healthcare system such as Kaiser

Permanente (KP), where doctors are salaried partners in a medical group. As a result, the emphasis switches to giving patients high-quality, reasonably priced care with a focus on illness prevention. In KP, there is a general organizational motive to support patients in leading healthy lives. Attention and resources can be directed toward the individuals who need medical attention when patients only seek care for preventive services.

Yet, doctors still struggle to effectively integrate dietary and lifestyle advice into their KP practices. Over the course of my two decades as a family doctor, the focus of medicine has shifted from treating acute, episodic conditions to managing chronic illnesses like obesity, diabetes, and hypertension over the long term. Even with the best of intentions, doctors sometimes feel that there is little we can do to improve or maintain the health of our patients, which lowers our sense of personal achievement. Furthermore, there is little incentive or reward for doctors to take the time to counsel, educate, or help patients adopt a healthier lifestyle, and quality metrics for chronic disease care inadvertently encourage doctors to aggressively prescribe multiple medications for conditions like diabetes and hypertension. These difficulties are having an impact on physician well-being and are a contributing factor to the depersonalization and emotional tiredness that characterize burnout, along with the rise in administrative and clerical duties. I just realized that in order to help deal with my burnout, I needed to make a crucial decision. I questioned myself:

Do I want to work as a healer or a drug "dealer" for the rest of my life? My career choice is healing. When you help patients regain their health and overcome chronic illnesses instead of just treating them with drugs, there is no greater delight in medicine. The appreciation I get from patients who change their lives serves as a constant reminder of why I decided to become a doctor. Having worked in professional settings for many years, I firmly believe that no medication or medical treatment can assist people in achieving better health than a prescription for a whole-food, plant-based diet, and active lifestyle.

PART 11

Chapter 3

The Optimal Macronutrient Ratio to Reduce Weight

Your body needs macronutrients carbohydrates, lipids, and proteins in huge quantities. According to a study, eating habits may have a greater impact on weight loss than dietary intake of carbohydrates, fats, and proteins.

Macronutrient counting has been a recent fad in weight loss.

These are the nutrients carbs, lipids, and proteins that your body needs in substantial quantities for proper growth and development. Conversely, micronutrients such as vitamins and minerals are those that your body only needs in trace amounts. While calculating calories and macronutrients are similar, macronutrient counting takes into account the source of calories. This article discusses why diet quality is important and what the ideal macronutrient ratio is for losing weight. For fat loss, calorie intake is more important than the ratio of macronutrients.

The quantity of food you eat has a greater impact on fat, carbohydrates, and protein content when it comes to fat loss. Among 600 overweight participants were randomized to a low-fat or low-carb diet throughout the course of a year-long trial. The low-fat diet group consumed 20 grams of fat per day and the low-carb group consumed 20 grams of carbohydrates per day over the first two months of the trial. Following a two-month period, participants in both groups started reintroducing either fats or carbohydrates into their diets until they achieved the lowest quantity they thought they could sustain.

Both groups cut their daily caloric intake by an average of 500–600 calories, although neither group was required to eat a certain amount of calories. The low-carb group dropped 13.2 pounds (6 kg) at the conclusion of the research, whereas the low-fat diet group lost 11.7 pounds (5.3 kg)—a difference of only 1.5 pounds (0.7 kg) over a year. In a different research, 645 overweight individuals were randomized to receive different amounts of fat (40% vs. 20%), carbohydrates (35% vs. 65%), and protein (25% vs. 15%) in their diets. Over the course of two years, all diets were similarly successful in inducing identical levels of weight reduction, regardless of the macronutrient ratio.

These and other findings demonstrate that, over time, any diet with fewer calories may result in comparable levels of weight reduction.

The Significance of Macronutrients

Every kind of macronutrient has a crucial function in maintaining the body's health. People usually need a mix of macronutrients for optimal health.

Carbohydrate

Many bodily tissues prefer the energy that carbohydrates provide, and the brain uses them primarily. Glucose, which enters the body's cells through circulation and enables them to operate, is produced by the body from carbs. During vigorous exercise, muscular contraction depends on carbohydrates. Carbohydrates help the body carry out essential tasks, such as digesting meals and regulating body temperature and heart rate, even while it is at rest.

Protein

Long chains of molecules known as amino acids make up protein. For bodily tissues to grow, develop, mend, and maintain themselves, these are vital. Every bodily cell contains protein, and maintaining the health of the muscles, bones, and tissues depends on consuming enough of it. Protein is also essential for many other biological activities, including immune system support, metabolic reactions, and cell construction and support.

Fats

An essential component of a healthy diet, fats can give the body energy. Dietary fats are an integral component of the diet and are involved in the creation of hormones, cell growth, energy storage, and the absorption of critical vitamins, even if some types may be healthier than others.

Dietary fiber: A vital component of a balanced diet

The Amount To Eat

The following macronutrient percentages are recommended by the federal Acceptable Macronutrient Distribution Range for maintaining good health and supplying necessary nutrition:

45–65% of the calories

15-20% fat

35% to 10% protein

Similar recommendations are made by the Dietary Guidelines for Americans, 2020–2025, which also acknowledges that individual differences in age, sex, and pregnancy status can affect an individual's calorie and macronutrient requirements. Furthermore, the following other variables may also have an impact on an individual's macro requirements:

Current fitness and weight objectives

Current medical conditions

Present-day muscular mass

Consume more fiber. Most likely, you've heard it before.

Chapter 4

But Why Is Fiber So Beneficial To Your Health?

The most well-known benefit of dietary fiber, which is mostly present in fruits, vegetables, whole grains, and legumes, is undoubtedly its capacity to either prevent or treat constipation. However, eating foods high in fiber can also help you maintain a healthy weight and reduce your risk of developing diabetes, heart disease, and some types of cancer.

It's not hard to choose appetizing foods that are high in fiber. Learn what foods contain dietary fiber, how much you need, and how to incorporate it into your meals and snacks.

What Does Food Fiber Mean?

Dietary fiber, roughage, or bulk are terms used to describe the parts of plant meals that are indigestible. Unlike other meal components like fats, proteins, or carbohydrates, which your body absorbs and processes, fiber is not metabolized by the body.

Instead, it passes mostly unharmed out of your body through your stomach, small intestine, and colon. Sometimes, fiber is separated into two groups: insoluble fiber and soluble fiber.

Soluble fiber dissolves in water. Absorbable thread. When this type of fiber dissolves in water, it forms a gel-like material. It can help reduce cholesterol and blood sugar levels. Foods high in soluble fiber include oats, peas, beans, carrots, citrus fruits, apples, barley, and psyllium. The insoluble thread; This kind of fiber helps pass material through the digestive system and increases stool volume, so it may be helpful for those who have constipation or irregular stools. Insoluble fiber can be found in whole-wheat flour, wheat bran, nuts, beans, and vegetables like potatoes, green beans, and cauliflower.

The proportion of soluble and insoluble fiber in various plant diets varies. Consume a wide range of high-fiber foods to get the most health benefits.

Advantages of a diet rich in fiber

A diet rich in fiber: restores regular bowel motions. Dietary fiber softens and makes your feces heavier and bigger. Because a thick stool is easier to pass, constipation is less likely to occur. Because fiber absorbs water and gives stool volume, it may assist in stabilizing loose, watery stools.

keeps the bowels healthy. Eating a diet rich in fiber may reduce the chance of hemorrhoids and colony-forming tiny pouches (diverticular illness). A high-fiber diet is also thought to reduce the incidence of colorectal cancer, according to studies. In the colon, some fiber is fermented. Scholars are investigating the potential function of this in averting colon illnesses. Cuts down on cholesterol. Low-density lipoprotein, or "bad," cholesterol levels can be lowered by soluble fiber, which is present in beans, oats, flaxseed, and oat bran. This can help reduce overall blood cholesterol levels. Additionally, research has indicated that eating foods high in fiber may lower blood pressure and inflammation, among other heart-healthy advantages.

Aids in blood sugar regulation. Fiber, especially soluble fiber, can assist lower blood sugar levels in diabetics by slowing the absorption of sugar. Insoluble fiber from a balanced diet may help lower the chance of type 2 diabetes.

Helps one reach a healthy weight. Because high-fiber foods are typically more filling than low-fiber foods, you'll probably eat less and feel fuller for longer. Furthermore, meals high in fiber typically require more time to consume and are less "energy dense," meaning they contain fewer calories per unit of food. prolongs your life. Research indicates that consuming more dietary fiber, particularly from cereals, may lower your chance of dying from all types of cancer and cardiovascular disease.

Your ideal selections for fiber

You might need to increase your intake of fiber if you're not receiving enough of it every day. Good options consist of:

Entire-grain goods

Berries

The veggies

Legumes, such as beans and peas

Seeds And Nuts

Foods that have been refined or processed, such as non-whole-grain cereals, pulp-free juices, canned fruits and vegetables, and white bread and pasta, have less fiber. Grain refining reduces the amount of fiber in the grain by removing the outer coat, or bran. After processing, some iron and B vitamins are added back to enriched meals, but not the fiber. foods and supplements enriched with fiber

In general, whole foods are preferable to fiber supplements. Supplements containing fiber, such as Metamucil, Citrucel, and FiberCon, don't offer the same range of fibers, vitamins, minerals, and other healthy components as whole foods.

Eating foods that have fiber added, such as granola bars, ice cream, yogurt, and cereal, is another approach to increase your intake of fiber. Usually, the extra fiber is identified by the terms "inulin" or "chicory root." Some people report feeling bloated after consuming foods high in fiber.

However, if dietary modifications are insufficient or if a person has certain medical issues like constipation, diarrhea, or irritable bowel syndrome, they might still require a fiber supplement. Consult your physician before using fiber supplements.

PART 111

Chapter 5

The Power of Plants: Comprehending Diets High In Plants

Is a plant-based diet synonymous with a vegetarian or vegan diet? Or does this diet merely require you to try to include more vegetables in your meals?

All of the aforementioned explanations are accurate in theory. "A vegan diet is sometimes referred to as a 'plant-based diet," explains Summer Yule, RD, a dietitian in Hartford, Connecticut. "Some people may use the term 'plant-based' to refer to diets that consist primarily, but not exclusively, of plant foods, and others may use it more broadly to refer to all vegetarian diets.

The Function of a Plant-Based Diet

Making plant-based foods the main component of your meals is the objective, "a plant-based diet limits foods like meats, dairy, and eggs and emphasizes foods like fruits, vegetables, and beans." Afterward, more limitations could be imposed based on your desired level of strictness.

"Depending on how each person understands it, it might exclude certain meals from animals entirely or only restrict consumption.

According to Harvard Health Publishing, this means that meat and fish don't necessarily have to be off-limits; you might just choose to consume them less frequently.

Chapter 6

Different Plant-Based Diet Types

Consider the term "plant-based" as a general term that encompasses other more specialized diets. For instance, although it includes fish and poultry, the Mediterranean diet emphasizes plant-based foods, making it a plant-based diet.

Among the plant-based diets are:

- Vegetable

- Detox

- Vegetarian Pesco

- Flexitarian or semi-vegetarian

- Vegetarian ovo

- Vegetarian Lacto

- Vegan lacto-ovo

Raw veganism

The well-liked Whole30 diet and lifestyle regimen are typically ineligible.

"While it is possible to follow the Whole30 diet entirely on plant-based foods, the traditional Whole30 diet places a greater emphasis on animal proteins.

Potential Advantages of a Plant-Based Diet for Health

Research published in the May 2017 Journal of Geriatric Cardiology states that the largest predictor of early death in the United States is having a poor-quality diet. When it comes to health and longevity, a traditional American diet heavy in processed meat, sodium, saturated and trans fats, and other unhealthy foods puts you at a disadvantage.

On the other hand, a diet that emphasizes whole foods and plant-based nutrients seems to have the opposite effect. In fact, the majority of those who follow this eating pattern do so because they believe it may have health advantages. " According to several research, eating a plant-based diet may lower your risk of acquiring [type 2] diabetes and improve reproductive characteristics. "There have been many cardiac benefits linked to eating this way, like reduced cholesterol," the Academy of Nutrition and Dietetics noted in a 2016 position paper. " Everyone can safely follow a well-planned plant-based diet, including young children, expectant mothers, and other caregivers."

A plant-based diet may help lower your risk of medication use, obesity, and high blood pressure, and may even help prevent or manage type 2 diabetes and heart disease, according to the study shown here. Here are some potential advantages of a plant-based diet in more detail.

The Key Ingredients in Raw Vegan Food

Raw vegan cuisine emphasizes eating foods in their uncooked, natural state and is founded on the idea of a plant-based diet. Without requiring any cooking, this diet highlights the vivid tastes, textures, and hues of fruits, vegetables, nuts, seeds, and grains. The end product is a wide variety of vibrantly colored foods that are high in vital nutrients and vivacious energy.

Chapter 7

The Advantages of Raw Vegan Food for Health

Sufficient in Nutrients:

Raw vegan dishes are high in dietary fiber, vitamins, minerals, and antioxidants. Eating a range of unprocessed plant-based foods offers a spectrum of nutrients that promote general well-being.

Digestive Wellness: Live enzymes included in raw vegan diets facilitate better digestion. These digestive enzymes aid in the breakdown of food, facilitate nutrient absorption and preserve digestive health.

Weight management: Raw vegan dishes' inherent low-calorie content will help you achieve your weight loss objectives. Meals high in nutrients satisfy your hunger while providing fewer calories than processed ones.

Bright Skin and Hair: Raw vegan diets are rich in vitamins, minerals, and antioxidants that support healthy skin and hair and give you a natural glow.

Enhanced Energy: Many people who switch to a raw vegan diet report feeling more energized. A diet high in complete, unprocessed meals promotes continuous energy production all day.

Innovative Cooking in Raw Vegan Cuisine

Vibrant Creations: Raw vegan dishes beautifully capture the spectrum of colors found in nature. The vivid colors of fruits, vegetables, and herbs enhance any dish's aesthetic appeal.

Creative Recipes: Making raw vegan meals inspires creativity in the kitchen. The options are unlimited, ranging from creamy nut-based sauces to noodles made with zucchini.

Fresh and Flavorful: Raw ingredients keep their inherent flavors, letting you enjoy each ingredient's essence in its purest form.

Diverse Textures: Raw vegan meals provide a pleasing sensory experience with a range of textures, from creamy smoothies to crunchy salads.

Quick and Convenient: Raw vegan meals are frequently quick to prepare, which makes them a great option for people with hectic schedules.

Chapter 8

Can You Lose Weight on a Plant-Based Diet?

While there are many reasons to switch to a plant-based diet, such as a lower chance of developing chronic illnesses and a smaller carbon imprint, losing weight can be another goal. Thankfully, a plant-based diet can also be beneficial in this regard. An analysis of vegan and vegetarian diets suggests that these eating habits may offer a healthier and more sustainable means of preventing overweight and obesity than other diets. Numerous studies linking plant-based diets to weight loss are cited in the same review.

One meta-analysis, for instance, examined 12 studies and found that those who were randomized to a plant-based diet lost almost 4.5 pounds more than those who followed a different, non-plant-based diet.

Plant-based diets, as noted by the Physicians Committee for Responsible Medicine, may facilitate weight loss since they emphasize whole meals, which are high in satisfying fiber.

Furthermore, since 1 gram (g) of fat contains 9 calories, compared to 1g of carbohydrates, restricting or avoiding higher-fat items, such as meat, may help you reach your weight objectives. Reducing calories could help you lose weight.

Chapter 9

Is Eating a Plant-Based Diet Bad for You?

It's probably not going to be enough to just stick to plant-based diets; you'll need to be mindful of the quality of the foods you're eating because many unhealthy items, like french fries and potato chips, can be classified as plant-based. Consuming unhealthy plant-based foods will raise your chance of gaining weight and developing diseases like heart disease. Another thing to consider is that you can experience diarrhea, constipation, or an increase in bowel motions when you first transition to a plant-based diet. This is because a lot of plant-based foods are high in fiber, which helps regulate bowel movements.

To give your body time to adjust, try adding more plant-based foods to your diet gradually. Also, make sure to stay hydrated both during and after the shift to a more plant-based diet. A plant-based diet will, for the most part, fulfill all of the major nutrient requirements.

Because so many fruits and vegetables are usually consumed, a well-planned plant-based diet can be nutritionally sufficient and especially rich in fiber, vitamin A, vitamin C, and potassium. That being said, you may need to monitor your levels of choline and vitamin B12 if you choose to go all-plant and abstain from animal products. "Animal sources are the main source of vitamin B12, and the finest sources of choline are liver and egg yolks. "A person might not be getting enough of these nutrients if they are avoiding animal products.

Chapter 10

Food Items In Plant-Bases Diet

When making the switch to a plant-based diet, people should concentrate on consuming the following food groups:

People who follow plant-based diets can eat all types of fruit. A plant-based diet includes all fruits, such as:

• Berries

• Fruits of citrus

• Papayas

• pears

• berries

• Honeydew

The avocado

The Veggies

Vegetables make up a large portion of a plant-based diet. Consuming a diverse selection of vibrant veggies offers an abundance of vitamins and minerals.

Some instances are:

• Brussels

4. Kale

• Carrots

• Vegetable

• Aubergine

The carrots

• Cucumbers

• Pickles

• carrots

Vitamins and carbs can both be found in plenty of root vegetables. They consist of:

• **The sweet potato**

1. potatoes

• Sugar plum squash

• Celery

Plantain

Legumes are an excellent source of fiber and plant-based protein. A person's diet might consist of a wide range of items, such as:

• Split peas

• Legumes

2. Peas

Beans, kidney

• Cocoa beans

Plants

Seeds make a delicious snack or a simple way to top off a soup or salad with extra nutrition. Sunflower seeds are an excellent source of vitamin E, and sesame seeds include calcium.

Other seeds consist of:

The pumpkin

Chia

hemp

Relax

Nuts

Nuts are a good source of vitamins, including vitamin E and selenium, and plant-based protein.

• Portugal

• Hazelnuts

• Cascabels

• Canes

• Mackerel

• Happatis

Wholesome Fats

Consuming omega-3 fatty acids and polyunsaturated and monounsaturated fats is essential.

Sources made from plants include:

• attorneys

• Almonds

• Chia grains

• Seeds of hemp

The flaxseed

The olive oil

• Canola seed

Whole Grains

In addition to being a great source of fiber, whole grains support stable blood sugar levels. They also include selenium, copper, and magnesium, among other necessary elements.

Whole grains consist of, for instance:

The brown rice

• Grats

- typed

- Raw wheat

Quinoa

- All-purpose bread

  Rye

- Gratley

Vegetarian Milk

There is a large selection of plant-based milk available in grocery stores and online for those who wish to cut back on dairy. These consist of:

2. Almond

- Hey

The coconut

- grain

- Grat

3. hemp

Just be careful to select plant milk options that aren't sweetened.

Chapter 11

Avoidable Foods

Merely cutting back on or giving up animal products does not imply that a plant-based diet is healthy. Additionally, it's critical to limit or stay away from unhealthy meals like:

• Canned goods

• sweet dishes like pastries, cakes, and biscuits

• refined white-type carbs

• processed substitutes for meat and vegetables that could be high in sugar or salt

• Too much salt

• meals that are deep-fried, oily, or fatty

recipes to get you going.

A person looking to start a plant-based diet can benefit from the following recipes:

Morning

• Baked oatmeal with apples and cinnamon

• Smoothie with almonds, wild blueberries, and flax

• Tofu Stir-Fry

Lunch.

• Salad of Tuscan beans

• Soup with butternut squash

• Roasted veggies with rosemary balsamic glaze

Supper

• Salad quinoa

Pizza with cauliflower

• Chili without meat

Final Course

- apricot-almond sauced apples

- figs coated in black chocolate

- Energy bites with peanut butter cups

A snack

- Banana protein bars with peanut butter

- Simple hummus

Kale chips with salt and cinnamon

Chapter 12

Seven-Day Menu for a Typical Plant-Based Diet

Day 1.

Omelette with tofu scramble

Lunchtime Cauliflower Rice Bowl topped with salsa, avocado, black beans, and corn

Dinner Pizza with veggies on top

Munchies: Zucchini chips

Day Two

Breakfast Muffins made with oatmeal

Lunch would be oyster crackers and tomato basil soup.

The supper is stir-fried veggies with tofu.

Munchies: Hummus wrap

Day Three

Oatmeal homemade bars for breakfast

Greek salad for lunch, together with a whole-grain pita bread slice

Kale and tofu curry for dinner

Eat berries and cashew yogurt with a dollop of peanut butter for a snack.

Day Four

Breakfast tortilla topped with salsa, peppers, and eggs

A side salad and a veggie burger for lunch

Dinner is roasted sweet potato fries and cauliflower "steak."

Snack: Hummus-topped vegetables

Day Five

Breakfast yogurt without dairy topped with oats and berries

Lunch is a tomato sandwich with pesto and olive oil drizzled on top.

Dinner is roasted tomatoes and whole-wheat pasta.

Snack: Roasted lentils

Day Six

Chia seed pudding for breakfast served with a tablespoon of almond butter and fresh fruit

For lunch, avocado toast

Dinner Enchiladas with vegan mushrooms

A handful of almonds for a snack

Day Seven

oatmeal for breakfast with almond milk

Quinoa bowl for lunch with sweet potatoes and roasted carrots

Dinner is a vegetarian chili with avocado slices on top.

Snack: Peanut butter on whole-wheat bread

Five Pointers for Newbies to Plant-Based Diets

Feeling overpowered because switching to a plant-based diet would mean completely changing your existing diet? Avoid overanalyzing it. Here, we provide five pointers for navigating the change.

1. Consider Alternatives to the Produce Aisle

To save yourself from having to shop every few days, stock up on grains, canned beans, and frozen or canned fruits and vegetables.

2. Replace Meat with High-Protein Vegetables

Among your many alternatives are chickpeas, pinto beans, tofu, tempeh, black beans, and dried peas. Additionally, you can select other high-protein foods, such as seitan and plant-based protein powder.

3. Ask the Waiter for Suggestions When Eating Out

In situations where the menu does not have a plant-based main course, a waitress may assist you in assembling a meal by providing sides and appetizers.

4. Select Cost-Effective Solutions

Buy produce that is in season and limit your diet to simple plant-based items like grains, beans, and frozen, and canned goods to keep grocery bills low.

5. Remember the Basics of Nutrition

At home, cook with less sugar, fat, and processed grains. These components can easily make a plant-based dinner prepared at home unhealthy.

SUMMARY

One thing that all plant-based diets have in common is that they exclude animal-derived meals in favor of plants. Vegetables, fruits, and whole grains take center stage in a diet rather than meat and dairy products. It's a tasty, healthful way to eat that has been demonstrated to offer major advantages for illness prevention and weight loss.

In society, physicians continue to have a position of trust. We have to work hard every day to keep earning and deserving of this trust. As a family physician, my work is not flawless every day. Some patients have little interest in altering their diet and way of life. But adopting lifestyle medicine, especially a plant-based diet has significantly enhanced my wellness, my patients' health, and my sense of contentment and fulfillment as a doctor. These days, I leave the clinic knowing that I did everything in my ability to provide my patients with the tools they need to take charge of their health.

In retrospect, I am immensely appreciative of Mr. Robert Park and his family. Had it not been for them, I might not have realized that a plant-based, whole-food diet is an effective means of achieving optimal health and well-being and is a key component of the solution to health, medical treatment, and physician wellness. Mr. Park could never have predicted how his life and death would affect me, and his legacy continues to this day with every patient I have the honor to care for.

www.ingramcontent.com/pod-product-compliance
Lightning Source LLC
Chambersburg PA
CBHW071109260726

48661CB00006B/2550